# Cubicle Cardio

## *The 1-Minute Workout Principle*

*Calories contain an inertia*

*It's when you cave into calories*

*That your diet and health take a beating.*

*This book hopes to provide basics to help you beat back.*

Written by

## Brian Shell

2

## Introductory Quote:

(By: Brian Shell)

*"If it wasn't work...*

*... they wouldn't call it workin' out."*

# CC = Cubicle Cardio

**(The 1-Minute Workout Principle)**

## CC Table of Contents:

## *Chapter Titles:*

## _Acknowledgements and Dedication_

First, I'd like to thank <u>all</u> the people who create an environment which enables a positive osmosis to occur. It is a conducive atmosphere of people trying to be better that leads to an overall achievement of other goals in ancillary avenues of our lives too. Thank you.

Second, I'm grateful to my mother. Love you Mom... always have... always will.

Finally, I dedicate this book to R.K. – you <u>Embody</u> and <u>Define</u> - - - _"Conquestuous."_

## 6
## _Disclaimer_

The author, Brian Shell, does not possess any degrees in exercise physiology or nutrition. The advice he communicates in this book are opinion, techniques, and observations he's made in over 30 years of playing amateur sports as well as own his exercise regimen's trials and errors. They are not meant to be communicated as a professional trainer's certified expertise… merely, a person who hopes to help you achieve your body appearance and exercise goals with a healthy dose of common sense tactics.

### *Initial Scenario*

Exercise. Consistency. Momentum.
Mindfulness. Results. Seated. Standing.

Little did I know 20 years ago when I was a
cubicle-crawling darkened-computer-room
engineer that Life was preparing me to write a
book about consciously achieving fitness
goals in the nooks and crannies of a hectic
corporate workplace environment.

Being that the corporation I worked for
seemed to have an endless array of birthday
celebrations, complete with cake and ice
cream, and the aroma of microwave buttery
popcorn emanating out of *someone's* office
every afternoon, it soon becomes evident that
taking the elevator to every meeting's
destination might not be your best bet health-
wise.

Also, as a formerly obese child in elementary
school, long-run habits need to be as positive
as possible so long-term health remains
consistent and strong.

Imagine a person of high responsibility. How
do they fit in fitness for any typical day?

Another example comes in terms of New
Years' resolutions. Two reasons people list

why they slack off from their health club attendance is *lack of time* and *inconvenience.*

Thus, 20 year later, this book was born. It was Life's preparation with "*wax on, wax off*" memory and ripples which enable these words of wisdom to flow for a new Healthy You.

Every journey begins with a single step.

Those simple steps <u>do</u> add up.

Let this book be yours.

Fit Happens!

Let it happen to You.

## CC = Cubicle Cardio

60 1-Minute Mini-Rodeos each Day

## *Chapter Zero*

*Be mindful and know your goals…*

Change doesn't happen by chance.

Prior to even beginning this book, I want you ask yourself about your health goals… your fitness goals… and your overall personal appearance goals.

The reason I write this is that if you don't know what your goals are in setting upon a lifetime fitness marathon, how you will you when you've arrived and if they're achieved?

It's a legitimate set of questions… because my approach is much different than others.

It's a *Life is a Marathon, Not a Sprint… Smarter, Rather than Harder* approach and overall attitude.

It's a *be willing to surrender a few battles in order to win the war* way of thinking about Life… especially when it comes to your overall fitness. Since all sports are filled with many clichés, here are a few more that apply: I present *a spoonful of sugar to help the medicine go down* exercise mindfulness and *a few steps back to make many leaps forward* mindset. But before all the talk about exercise, you need to know your goal.

When I played competitive racquetball, my goal was cardiovascular endurance. Many opponents I played had more sheer talent than me, but because I wanted to win more and was in better shape, I often beat them in tie-breakers because my fitness was superior.

Likewise, when I go to the gym, I lift very <u>light</u> weights <u>many</u> times with <u>many</u> sets because I'm going for tone instead of going for hulking muscle mass like a lot of the body-builders next to me. My goal is not going for size; I'm going for shape. Thus, I exercise appropriately for the goal of not growing out of the nice suits I've purchased... because my tailor has taken me to task on it and told me, "*I can take your pants in and out all day long, but I can't take the shoulders out of your suit coat if you get too buff.*"

Thus, this book is all about **being Mindful**. Know your Goal so you know when you Arrive. Then set your next set of goals with the new view of You.

### *Two Exercise-Free Months… then Back to the Gym – Lessons Learned*

From June thru July of 2013, I ran an experiment… to stay exercise-free for two months.

No Gym.  No Vitamins.  No Stretching.  No Yoga.  No Weights.  No Diet either.

In other words, I took a much-needed breather.  It was nice.  Very nice.

What did I learn?

Before anything else, it was nice to let everything heal.

All my muscle tweaks, sore joints, and strained body aches took ample time to recover.  I allowed them more than their due time.  The funny thing is that atrophy did set in a bit.

Initially, I learned that the inertia needed to jump back into the exercise saddle got steeper the longer I disciplinedly decided to stay away.  It was tough to *not* exercise – period – on purpose – especially when it had been such a standard staple of my life for the past few years… and then during the years in my 20's when I used to play professional racquetball. Before I decided to rejoin my old gym, after 2 months of no stretches, I finally allowed myself a night of deep yoga out underneath the stars. It felt majestic. And the one thing I didn't expect… was that during that night I felt an Emergence.

What I didn't realize is that those two months away actually promoted new growth – BETTER – than I was growing when I was working out almost everyday.

Healing does need to happen.

It's like a sculptor putting more clay on his masterpiece and tryin' to figure what to do next. It gave it a chance to Breathe. Allow the paint to dry. There's a line from the movie *City Slickers* that I quote often where ol' Jack Palance tells Billy Crystal and his friends, "*You city slickers… you spend 50 weeks a year putting knots in your rope, and then you expect that all you need is 2 weeks away to untie 'em.*"

That is *so* True. Our bodies need that downtime.

If they're always On, what do we do to turn them Off?

Also though, there were times during those 2 months away that I couldn't have done what I did with*out* being away from the gym. That's the thing a lot of doctors don't tell you. The exercise routine does sap a certain level of energy and creative spark from your psyche – right off the top. Example: During the 2013 Fourth of July holiday weekend in Traverse City, MI… due to all the hotel rooms being booked up on a Friday night (July 5$^{th}$) I needed to drive over 25 hours without sleep in order to find a room. I could *not* have done that if I'd been working out in the gym in my normal exercise routine. My body would have been too tired, sore, and sapped of energy to drive all those 800 miles that day – searching for a safe place to sleep where I wouldn't get in trespassing trouble. I even joked with a sheriff's deputy at 2 a.m. in front of a 7-Eleven: *"I'm joking when I say this officer, but… Please, book me. It'd be easier to get a bed for the night."* He laughed. He understood. A packed 4$^{th}$ of July weekend makes vacancies rare.

The point is: Sometimes, taking a break from the exercise is, in fact - <u>Necessary</u>.

The issue then becomes maximizing such vacations-from-exercise wisely.

For me, I arranged my time-away to line up with vacation and meetings.

Also, June and July are some jim-dandy **fine** months to savor. Though being in the dog-days of summer – they *are* hot & humid. That's when heat-exhaustion can sap and tapout a routine quick. So ultimately, adding the silences helped make my music flow.

In returning to my exercise routine though, my number one priority was doing so - slow.

That way, my muscles and joints could ease back into the grind. Old injuries are like rust – their aching never sleeps. So letting the muscles around those creaky hip and knee joints atrophy only made getting back into the routine tougher.

The typical gym gossip, chit-chat, and cliques still exist, but now, I see them from a fresh perspective, a bit new, and rejuvenated. I embrace seeing old friends. Noticing who was diligent in achieving their exercise goals and those who had slacked off was an unexpected bonus. Those who over-achieved re-stoked my inspiration to train – **Hard.** They reignited the drive and the desire to put in the work necessary to look good… and it *is* work… *hard work.* But it's worth it when the results start to re-emerge. The inner smile you re-start to wear warms you. It helps keep you going. It refuels the fire inside.

Another cool thing about taking some time away is that it gave my muscles a chance to take a break from the normal routine I'd taken them through; thus, coming back is like a nice confusion for those muscles… which helps them grow. If they get used to what you do to exercise, the efficiency of your training sessions suffers. Their senses get dulled.

That's why a lot of trainers recommend maximum intensity interval training… so you shock the muscles into growth. While that works, I like the more natural way… taking a nice break… enjoying my time away… maximizing the tasks that demand more creative juice & spark… and then coming back *wanting* to do it… instead of feeling like I *have* to do it… all because I'd gotten dulled to the grind. Pace yourself for Life's Marathon.

That's a huge difference in training attitudes – <u>wanting</u> to do it instead of <u>having</u> to do it.

Recovery *does* take time. Ya can't cheat it.

Another ancillary benefit was that I took a disciplined approach to breaking old habits and interrupted many patterns. Then in coming back to such familiar routines, I took a different light to see if they still held water. Were they ultimately constructive or destructive to my overall goals and destination?

Knowing that you *can* make a change and break a habit once enables you to learn and *know* that you can *do it again* when called upon. That's a good knowledge to Know.

It helps in coming back too… because now, I haven't forgotten the routine… but tweak it to adjust to the changes I'd like to see made manifest. The choices I now make in how, when, and where I exercise are consciously different. Being conscious of *Being Conscious* is a good thing. *Being Conscious* about being <u>Health</u> <u>Conscious</u> is good too.

So put the "*earn*" in Learn. Learn how to be Health Conscious – consistently consistent.

Benefits abound by coming back to an organized gym. First, I really remembered how much I like having a lot of exercise equipment in one place. It helps me increase my efficiency, intensity, and balance. Second, I relearned, yet again, I can break through any wall of inertia set upon me if I focus my mind on it enough. Third, emergent growth is cool. Nuff' said. Fourth, as we grow and evolve, the reptilian metaphor… of shedding a skin so we don't suffocate inside the one we're in… applies. Growth requires growth.

One of my tailors noticed that I'd been working out. His quip dripped with snark: "*Great, none of **our** clothes will fit.*"

That's true. Ordinary clothes aren't made to fit the athlete. They fit ordinary folk.

Another tailor told me when getting larger slacks, *"Ah, yes sir, men's slacks have a way of shrinking over time."* It's nice when it goes the other way around… ripening nicely.

Such growth is a nice thing to achieve, and squeezing into ol' skinny jeans you couldn't let yourself throw away… and having them fit again after years away is f*ckin' cool… *Awesome!* It's like rediscovering an old best friend and then remembering how and why they became your favorites in the first place. Everyone has one. It's allowed. But then you also recognize and realize how the years have taken their toll to those ol' skinny jeans… and then extend its metaphor to the mileage you've put on your own body.

We stretch our seams. That's where we really need to take time to Heal.

But don't stay away too long. Reacquiring its *"Structure"* does take Time.

An old swami told me: *"Three days in one place… no cobwebs. Fourth day? Cobwebs."*

That's the Balance of knowing when to Return. After two months, the rust started creeping back. It never sleeps. But a breather is nice… needed… and <u>Necessary</u>.

## *Introduction*

I think one of the best things that happened to me recently was when I was on my way home about 20-22 months ago… it was a nice day, blues skies, not too hot, not too cold… and I just stared up at the big blue sky and thought aloud while driving:

*"I'm just gonna start trying harder from here on out… right now."*

Upon telling that decision to my Mom later in the day, a few tears came to my eyes when I made the resolution out loud.  It spoke my vow with *the Breath of the Eternal*.  I said it to the Universe.  It compelled me to Try… even when I am too weary.

It's a conscious choice really.

You either try harder or you don't.
You start to care more or you don't.
You do it right even when no one is looking.

And by buying this book, I <u>ask</u> you to do the same:

**Make a vow to Start Trying Harder - period.**

Be conscious about being health conscious

Prepare to be prepared

Try to try harder

It's like a train leaving the station... slow at first... then the momentum builds... yet overcoming that initial zero-inertia is often the hardest part.

So consider the following:

+ Disciplined inspiration
+ Re-establishing momentum
+ Think of exercise like brushing your teeth
+ Make a pact with yourself (and reward yourself)

Ya gotta wanna get better.
Ya gotta wanna try harder.

These days, we are inundated by ads for cosmetic surgery and that there's "*a pill for everything*" mentality which may often offer a temporary gain, but it doesn't solve and/or cure the root cause of bad choices... which have a habit of compounding over time.

In other words, you can't cheat your bad habits.
You have to reprogram them with good ones.

So put the cult in Culture – possess a *Cult of Personality*.
Develop a newfound *Cult of Exercise and Energy*.
It'll help you get your mojo back and workin'.

Often, I consider my **1-minute-workout** <u>concept</u> a *"stop and smell the roses"* philosophy towards taking care of your health – one minute at a time – at least 60 times a day.

Really, my *"One Minute Workout Principle"* is all about elevating your heart rate with a conscious mindfulness that gets away from the low-hanging-fruit mentality of always trying to find the closest parking space... of always taking the easy way out.

One of the reasons this is a passion of mine is that I was the fattest kid in my elementary school. I remember one day a kid came up to me and grabbed by tubby tummy and shouted, *"Pinch an inch? Damn, I can pinch a mile!"*

That was a low day.

And I've recognized that while I now have a *Lean & Mean* mentality these days, there's always a fat kid *inside* who loves to **gorge**... who is the consummate *Cookie Monster*... spinning the Roy Rogers quip - *"I've never met a chocolate chip cookie I didn't like."*

So knowing that, I've learned to <u>balance</u> the good with the bad... and to reward myself so I feed my soul with the foods the fat kid craves... while treating food as fuel with fruits and veggies as my new tools. That's

why I published my *"**Dessert First Diet**"*
book too.

It had *"Leave any room for dessert?"*
beginnings… and then reversed that
mentality… so you eat the foods you like
when you're the hungriest so they taste the
best… and then get back to work eating right.
It's like the camel who knows he must cross a
desert and thus fills his belly for that long
lonesome valley… but who rewards himself
after the Journey.

For me, my big change away from obesity
happened when I saw the movie *"Rocky"* for
the first time back in the late 1970's.  It
caused me to start to jog.  That exercise
connection continued upon going to college…
when I subscribed to *"Muscle & Fitness"* for
a year… with a *bucket list* item of getting the
vertical line down the center of my abs.

Then I added the complimentarity of Arnold
Schwarzenegger's *"Sculptor"* ideas from his
Mr. Olympia movie titled *"Pumping Iron"*
where you are the artist of your own body…
someone who sculpts and creates a living
work of Art – You!

So **Sculpt** a **Masterpiece** that would make
even Michelangelo **Mesmerized**.

Sometimes you only learn life's lessons by
going *through* tough times.

*Fat & Happy* vs. **Lean & Mean** – <u>Assertive Confidence</u> sells itself.

Those choices are yours… but in this book, I've tried to sway away from the "*Looks good from far… but is far from good*" sort of thing today's society's got going.

As ya gotta be just as good up-close-and-personal as from far-away.

That way when you step on the scale, you don't say *two words* that start with "*Oh*" and end with an exclamation point.  ;)

Don't settle for less than you deserve.
Assertive Dignity is a Decency we <u>all</u> Deserve.
A rose must grow through a lot of dirt to bloom.

**Bloom where you are planted**

So with all that said, on with the show…
…and remember, The Show Must Go On.

Everything counts One.
Make every One count.

## *Chapter One*

## *Premise*

*"Well... time ta get back to work."*

That's my mantra every day I hit - *the Gym.*

It's not <u>what</u> you do; it's <u>how</u> you do it.

Thus, *the Gym…* is a State of Mind.

It could even be your cubicle too.

As we embark on this **Cubicle Cardio** (CC) journey and its accompanying 1-minute-workout principles, I'd like to explain why I feel it works.

The thing is; you become **<u>Mindful</u>** at incorporating extra exercise into all the nooks and crannies of your day to boost your metabolism, and something important seeps in.

**You soon realize how much <u>Work</u> it takes to *Achieve* your physical fitness goals.**

Because of that *A-Ha moment*, you soon make many mini paradigm shifts in every aspect of your life so you don't feel like you're wasting your time with the exercise you do *Do*.

Ya can't cheat that.

**Weight is your body's Mirror.**

**It's 100% Truthful.**

**It never lies.**

Often it takes one right change in a crucial aspect of your life that helps rearrange your understanding of all the other aspects of your life. It's a *"pinch your pennies and the dollars will take care of themselves"* mentality. You start to care more. And since hard work is simply that – hard work – you realize that even if you're going in the wrong direction weight-wise, it's easier to steer back into the right direction simply because you have <u>momentum</u> and <u>consistency</u> that develop the overall goal's destination into reality.

Ask yourself: is it easier to change direction if you're in motion or at a complete stop?

The answer is that when you're already in motion, even in the wrong direction, the fact that you're moving helps you change course. Bodies in motion tend to stay in motion. That momentum is a good thing. Bodies at rest tend to stay at rest. So getting going makes a difference. Thus, if you work out *60 times a day for 1-minute at a time*, you become *conscious* and *mindful*. In doing so, you start to make better decisions regarding the food you buy and eat… realizing, if it's <u>not</u> in the home, chances are, it won't make it to your mouth.  Also, you start to buy and eat healthier foods too… simply because you start to treat food as fuel with fruits and veggies as your tools… an acquired taste.

And it's a poor workman who blames their tools.

The windmill principle… this is Lady Gaga's trainer's technique: Keep your windmill lightly slightly spinning… all throughout the day… instead of spinning it once a day for 60 minutes straight at the health club and then veggin' out with it at zero all day afterwards. It's an interesting idea, isn't it?

You want your metabolism's windmill spinning efficiently… all day long.

It reminds me of stoking the fire of a steam-train, with kindling… instead of throwing one big log on the fire which takes an eternity to start, stay lit, and burn long and deep.

Augment/supplement your normal workout with many mini-make-overs.

**Here are a few slogans for you I've seen along the way to fitness goals:**

"*Fit Happens*" – slogan in an Ann Arbor fitness boutique – Bodies in Balance

*"Set Goal. Accomplish. Repeat."* – D1
Detroit fitness boutique slogan

*"Concede that we will lose a few battles of the muffin-top bulge in order to win the lifelong weight loss war."*

*"Workout enough **to schvitz** but not enough to sweat while at work."*

*"How do you quit a bad habit? You make new friends."*

That's where joining a gym or a health club in order to overcome a past bad habit can help. Sometimes when we make a financial commitment to our health, it helps our fitness goals to manifest into reality… sooner rather than later. It jumpstarts your workout routine… so you fit exercise into your daily routine. Habit is replaced by habit.

It's when I make mistakes that I learn the most… simply because I don't want to be wrong again. So as Tavis Smiley says, *"Fail upwards."*

Today I was speaking with a fat 51 year old construction worker who was watching me work out in my yard… and came over to tell me how he used to be in great shape. I told him, "You can *still* get back in great shape." He replied, *"Well, I learned to eat over the past 25 years."* My thought afterwards is that so many people *can* do it (get back into shape); they just don't *think* that they can. That kind of *"can't do"* thinking has to change into a *"can do"* attitude. You *can* do it! All it takes is a minute at a time.

Carpe Diem/seize-the-day attitudes – fate is a function of choice - Yet like in *"Dead Poets Society,"* sucking the marrow out of life doesn't mean choking on the bone.

Now with those quotes and thoughts out of the way, let's mention a few definitions:

Adrift – rowing too many different oars only rows you in circles
Acquired tastes – rewards earned via hard work – perspective
Knowledge is the new wealth. Perspective is power.

Finally, here's a quote of mine I'd like to share to end this first chapter:

**Families who train together... remain together.**

Enough said. Now let's get down to the meat and potatoes of my Cubicle Cardio!

## *Chapter Two*

## *Consistency*

It's easier to reach the correct destination, even if you're now going in the wrong direction, than if you're not going at all... simply because of consistent momentum.

That's the problem I have with working out too hard. It causes muscle soreness that precipitates you taking a few days off to heal and for the muscles to grow. The problem then is getting the gumption to get back into the normal routine because you've broken your momentum's consistency. Do you see the conundrum? For example, I find that I write better when I don't work out. My workouts sap a certain creative energy it takes to sit down in a room all alone and just write. So my writing desire saps my workout desire. The price I pay is my waistline when I'm trying to finish a book... like this one. It breaks my desire to stay consistent with my exercise regimen so I can fuel my writing regimen.

Recently, I saw an obese woman taking a walk with her walker... "*At least she's trying.*" That was the first thought that came to mind. She was making a willful effort to curb her battle with her waistline. Sometimes that very first exercise jumpstarts it all into motion.

Everyone has choices. So make good, healthy choices… not bad ones.

There's always a quality vs. quantity battle that goes on – coupon incentives and their consequences of buying too much bulk food often saps your consistency. My advice is to savor quality over quantity because it feeds your soul to a finer degree and makes you enjoy your food. But this battle also goes on in the way you lift weights or exercise.

For example, high impact jogging vs. an elliptical cardio machine… one saves the knees.

How long does it take on a treadmill to work off your food and drink? That's another thing to consider in quality versus quantity. An example that comes to mind the price it costs to be a high-quality microbrew 6-pack versus a case of 24 cans of cheap beer. They're the same price. But with one purchase, you'll consume a lot more calories.

Balance and moderation in any endeavor is crucial for continued success.

The "*habit*" of exercise is one of the hardest to acquire in terms of lifelong consistency… life is a sinusoid… with ups and downs.

However, the momentum you gain when you see results in the mirror and on the scale is priceless. It refuels your desire to continue onwards with your exercising... even if it's just one minute at a time, 60 times a day.

As a testimony, when I am consistent with my workouts, my knee problems go away (I was consciously and actively strengthening the muscles around the knee), my wheezing (due to smoking) disappears so I breathe better, my intensity increases, my endurance soars... and my self-confidence makes me smile at myself in the mirror.

In watching an ad for chiropractic care yesterday, the thought that came to mind is that so many of us have our vertical center of gravity *away* from the line of our spine. If your big belly is pulling your back out of place... consider exercising it back to the correct anatomic position. Just like diabetes, some back pain (and even arthritis) can be cured by simply losing the extra weight your body has to carry around that wears out your joints... as well as strengthening the muscles around those joints that are sore for you. In those cases of arthritis, a major league baseball pitcher showed me (in person) that the way he rehabs his throwing shoulder is with a lot of very, very light weight, high-repetition exercises which strengthen all of the smaller muscles <u>inside</u> the shoulder joint. He advised that the big muscles on the outside are easy to build big, but it's the small muscles inside that actually attach to the joints which need not to be ignored either.

The moral of this chapter comes in the form of the question, *"How can we have time if we don't make time?"*

Noah started building the ark before it started to rain. The same applies with your body... an ounce of proactive prevention is worth a pound of cure.

Isaac Newton's First Law of Motion says: a body at rest tends to stay at rest... and a body in motion tends to stay in motion... unless an external force acts upon it for it to change.

Here's a poignant Powerhouse Gym quote from an email they sent that speaks volumes. Its title is "Successfully Achieving Goals" – *"First of all, you have to make a decision to START. You can say you're too busy, too tired, too (insert excuse), but how badly do you want it? You cannot achieve results without STARTING! Also, have you set a specific, written goal? Psychologists who study the art of success claim that 95-97% of people who do NOT have written goals fail, while the 3-5% who do have written goals triumph. You need to be among that elite 3-5% if you want to succeed! Are you making your fitness goals a priority in your life? We can all say we don't have enough time. And who does? But the bottom line is, determine what you value? Your health? Do you value productive energy when spending time with your family and/or kids? If these are true, than you cannot afford to NOT make the time. When you finally make exercise a priority, NOT an option, you'll begin to feel more energized and less stressed. And feel a sense of accomplishment that you are doing it"!*

Prolonged sustainability is the main key.
It takes momentum's maintenance.
It takes consistency.
You can do it.
Just START.

## *Chapter Three*

## *Food as Fuel*

"***Basic Fire Science***" – "The form of a solid or liquid fuel is an important factor in the ignition and burning rate. For example, a fine wood dust ignites easier and burns faster than a block of wood. Some flammable liquids, such as diesel oil, are difficult to ignite in a pool but can ignite readily and burn rapidly when in the form of a spray or mist."

The more muscle you build, the more calories it takes to maintain your current bodyweight… in other words, your muscles need more food to fuel them. This also means that if you consume the same amount of calories while gaining muscle, you'll start to lose weight as you get into shape because your body burns more fuel than it uses.

Therefore, frontload your calories from the beginning of the day… and taper off as evening approaches.

"*Broccoli doesn't brag.*" This is a quote I overheard from a guest on Dr. Oz. I thought you might like it. Dr. Oz certainly did.

Shopping around the edges of a grocery store… this is one way to keep the processed foods from entering your diet. In a sense, it's more of a Mediterranean diet because you consume fruits, veggies, proteins, dairy, cheeses, and yogurts. Notice the absence of carbohydrates though when you shop around the edges of the store. It's good for you.

Just the gist of *"The Zone Diet"* – food is the most powerful drug you will ever consume.

I love *"The Zone Diet"* and feel it works... which is one reason I recorded my song *"Eat Some Vegetables"* and my published my book *"Dessert First Diet."* I've learned a healthy approach to living that enables desserts to creep in to savor and enjoy.

There's an importance of drinking water when it comes to weight loss too... drink a few glasses of H2O before meals... it fills you up and helps you eat less calories when the food arrives. Also, it hydrates you with pure water which our bodies are made up of.

Sometimes, I also believe in the Camel Diet – where you fuel yourself fully to cross your desert before you are able to eat again after many, many hours of knowing you'll do without food. It's loading up for a long voyage type of thinking.

Then there's my Caveman Diet – which is good for my *"All Men Are Dogs"* book which preaches high protein intake... so we have the fuel to build the muscles we want.

Another interesting tidbit comes from Good Morning America where GMA's did blind taste tests of diet foods (such as Nutrisystem, Jenny Craig, Weight Watchers)... and one of the food critics said they all tasted *"synthetic."* The chef sitting beside him totally agreed with that assessment. None of them really liked the taste of the food... yet, the starving students were more accepting of it and actually liked the cheaper foods better than the gourmet food critics who seemed to like the more expensive varieties that were offered. I tend to agree. It tastes like fake food processed to make it low in calories. So weigh your shopping purchases well. You can do better just buying fresh foods.

Did you know: Skipping breakfast increases chances of obesity by 450% (this comes Men's Health magazine). It's an interesting tidbit that makes me hungry in the morning.

Another tidbit I was told by a personal trainer is that doing your cardio before weight lifting is wrong. The body needs to burn through sugar before it taps into fat. Weight lifting does this... which is why that trainer advises doing it first. Also though, weight lifting doesn't make you sweat as much as cardio... so getting on the weight machines is actually a cleaner prospect since you don't have to wipe off your sweat from the machines if you use them first.

Likewise, I advise to cure your hunger cravings with the tastiest foods first. You eat what you want when you're the hungriest... that way they taste the best... then get back to work eating right. It's my "*Dessert First Diet*" book's philosophy. That way, you nip your cravings in the bud before they blossom into a binge.

## *Chapter Four*

## *Cubicle Cardio*

Time is valuable.  If you don't have time for an hour at the gym, this exercise philosophy augments your workouts all through the day.

It's also about the intensity with which you workout.

Another thing to consider is using the mirror and video… just as much as the scale.  I think that taking a video of yourself dancing is probably the best way to analyze your body image… as motivation to work out and exercise more.  First, watch it alone.  Then, watch it with a friend by your side.  It's as if you see yourself from a different POV.

Destination Walking – Do you have an actual place you're going?  A true north?
Or are you just walking?  They say that if you have your goal in mind, you achieve it with better results than if you don't have a set goal on top of your consciousness.

One way to avoid the endless treadmill?
Always give priority to activities that serve the greatest purpose… walking with a destination in mind and a time to be there by.

Remember the little train that could: "*I can do this… I can do it!*"  Belief in oneself is a powerful tool to add. The thing to keep in mind is that everything counts. Even one minute of somehow raising your metabolism adds up… just as each calorie counts too.

So another thing about the Cubicle Cardio principle is working out at work without the messy sweat. That requires stoking your metabolism with focusing on what you can do. Also, it might help alleviate your 2 o'clock crash after lunch when a nap would be a blessing. For example… walking up stairs and taking the elevator down (to save your knees). Another one is doing isometric flexing while in your chair. Some people now have stand-up desks rather than being seated all day. Even taking a walk in place of some people's smoking break works too. Perhaps try taking a lap around the loop of offices before going to get a cup of coffee. Another one is doing small isometric abdominal crunches while you drive. Personally, my favorite exercise to do while waiting in line at a store is toe raises. That why, I continually improve my balance and the shape of my calves. You can do a few while waiting for the printer, at the Xerox machine, while cooking a meal… along with using the kitchen counter to do ballet stretches and mini-squats like a ballet dancer. They all add up.

The whole premise is to raise your heart rate ever so slightly… MANY TIMES A DAY…

instead of just once while at a gym. A nice metaphor to consider is that your heart rate and metabolism are like an airplane. If you do 60 1-minute workouts all throughout the day, your metabolism is then similar to being at cruising altitude rather than being grounded after one trip up in the air each day.

Another thing about this kind of approach to exercise is that it eliminates the crash that comes after a grueling workout. If you work out really hard, there's the need for recovery time after hitting the gym or health club for an hour. For example, I realize that if I work out early in the day, I don't have the same gumption to sit down and write the books that make up my portfolio of published material... 30 books so far. So balance in realizing I need a certain level of energy to write which a hard workout saps. Also, when I apply Cubicle Cardio one-minute-workouts while I write my books, I find that it gives me a nice mental breather where my mind tends to percolate on what I want to write next.

"*Excess within control*" is a great line from the film "*Somewhere in Time*" when it comes to this book and its philosophy.

Increasing your flexibility helps your blood-flow. So also consider adding basic stretching to your arsenal of one-minute-workouts. Also though, it makes you feel great! Yoga works. It does. My former boss used it to lose 30 pounds and 4 inches around his waist. Moreso though, I believe that it's made him more conscientious about his diet. That's because if you put a lot of time into making exercise a priority, there's a part of you that doesn't want to squander your gains by eating a donut or a slice of pizza.

If you've seen the impressive results from the P90X exercise infomercials, I'd read that its results are a direct result of the "*muscle confusion*" technique. What that means is changing up your routine often so that your muscles don't get in a rut. That's because once they get used to a stagnant routine done repeatedly; you don't get the same gains. So its premise is to switch up your workouts so your muscles never know what's coming next. In other words, it's like a freeform way of exercising so you never repeat yourself.

Isometrics & Kegels are prime ingredients of making up many small workouts throughout the day. The way it works is to 1) flex, 2) hold it, and 3) release. Then do this repeatedly at various times in the day.

A walk becomes a dance once you sing to it. This is what I've heard is Zumba's dancing premise. If you like the TV show "*Dancing with the Stars*," notice the dancers are all in such great shape. Dancing does that. Think about adding a dance or two to your day.

In other words, when in doubt, dance!

*"Drive for show, putt for dough"*… that's a slogan I recall from the golf course. Yet in a video golf game I once played, the game allows you to drive your swing *"into the red"* when swinging. It gives more power, but you sacrifice control when you *"go into the red."* It's the same way with exercise and training. Going into the red may get better and faster results, but that's when you risk the chance of injury. So moderation is key.

The whole point I want to reinforce is that my Cubicle Cardio techniques are to add it to supplement your normal workout at a gym or health club.

There are social aspects of joining a gym that you should be aware of too… as it can often be a *"Peyton Place"* – but it also fosters an environment where you surround yourself with people who promote healthy choices. So sometimes overhearing the petty gossip from those who work out in small groups can help and hurt simultaneously. It's one reason I've switched gyms more than once. Sometimes no judgment is a good thing.

Now here's an economics metaphor: Be the CEO of your own body. You can be bullish about your exercise or bearish and still achieve your goals, but pigs always lose.

While I walked on a treadmill, I read an exercise magazine mentioning a UK study showed that employees work 15% more efficiently the days they exercise. Food for thought as you consider adding exercise to the nooks and crannies of your day.

The whole point of cubicle cardio is that no one needs know you're workin' out at work. It's a *"No sweat, no pain, all gain"* kind of approach so you seize your reality daily.

It's about increasing your exercise mindfulness so you want to exercise... instead of feeling like you have to exercise. That's where taking a break can boost morale. It promotes muscle growth too because it allows for recovery time... both physical and mental. That's something you want to avoid... the burnout. Because that's when all of your gumption drops to absolute zero. As they say, it's easier to steer a ship going in the wrong direction as long as it's moving.

If you stop exercising all together for a long period of time, there becomes a mental hurdle that becomes hard to clear if you try to regain your past results all at once.

This is where Cubicle Cardio's philosophy to do many mini-workouts can regain pace and consistency. Getting going again is tough. When there are those days I don't want to workout, sometimes I force myself to go to

the gym and just walk on the treadmill. At
first, I resist it, but once you get used to it,
you're glad you did. Regaining momentum
of a regular routine is like any other habit, it
takes 28 days to become consistent. It
becomes a typical part of the day instead of
one salient blip. You don't want the extreme
blip. Instead, you want the area beneath the
Bell Curve. That's your exercise sweet spot.

Just remember that you're the only one who
can do the work. It helps if you want to do it.
Incorporating sixty one-minute-workouts all
throughout the day gains that mindfulness
momentum which soon turns into a typical
day's regimen and routine.

Now I'll finish up this chapter with a list... as
it seems like people love lists: 1) Exercise,
exercise, exercise – just start, 2) Time and
place – find that perfect place and treat it as
sacred ground, 3) Turn off and tune in – no
interruptions, 4) Use an outline – manageable
goals that can be achieved, 5) Set goals –
rituals which are doable, 6) Record your
progress – separate processes, 7) Take
necessary breaks, 8) once done start anew.

## *Chapter Five*

## *Spot Reductions*

At some point, I think even the most diligent exercise people throw their routine out the window… and then take a huge slide of "*not caring*." I've had those moments. I'm sure most people do. There was one period of time I purposely said, "*Screw calories*." Unfortunately, all my gains were lost due to it, but it served a purpose. I was burned out.

The problem, at the time, was that when I came back to working out, I thought I could just do a lot of abdominal exercises to regain my six-pack abs. It doesn't work like that. Think of seeing results as peeling layers off an onion. For example, when I did incorporate more fat-burning cardio to my routine, the progress caused a gain in gumption. Then, I noticed that I had to readjust my baseball caps. I thought, "*Boy, what a fat head I had!*" But that's the way it works, you don't lose in a spot. You lose weight all over… that's when the vascularity of your veins starts to show again. That's when you become proud of your abs and show them off.

There is a fallacy in a lot of TV ads and infomercials that try to sell spot reduction exercise equipment… such as for the abs.

Your body doesn't work that way. You see; you may get great abs but if you still have layers of fat covering them, you won't see them. Still though, sometimes the whole point is just to add that exercise equipment to an overall exercise routine which includes calorie-burning fat-busters. Until you take off the flab, you can't see the muscle those gadgets want you to build.

Then there's the TV claims: "*when dieting and exercise aren't enough*" – which is maybe when you're in denial as to the effort you're putting into your workouts and the real foods you're truly eating. One way to monitor this is starting a food diary… all those "*safe*" snacks and finger foods do add up… just like the person in the office with the candy bowl. Be a detective with a food diary. Each calorie you consume does count. For example, Dr. Oz mentioned a woman who went on a fruit diet, but because she ate too much fruit, she actually gained weight… no matter how nutritious her diet was… simply because she consumed more calories each day than her body was able to burn off. At the end of the day, what matters is the balancing scale of calories in versus calories out. If you take in more calories than your body burns in a day, you will gain weight – period.

So trim the fat in the food you eat, and then have fun

My philosophy for kicking a habit is doing
*"one last hurrah"* to celebrate *"the damage
done"* and then move on to a new chapter of
Life… with no regrets or what ifs.
Sometimes the signposts and turning points in
our life need one final celebration. It's kind
of like a New Years Eve kind of thinking to
achieve new goals. As a matter of fact, I
heard of a joke about a new gym called
*"Resolutions"* that is a health club in January
but turns into a bar for the remaining eleven
months of the year. Sadly, it's too true.

I've also heard that the more time you spend
in a store, the more you tend to spend. Also,
if you bring home food, you tend to eat it…
so consider more single-serving sized bags
instead of bringing home bigger bags of
supersized treats… as it's a lot easier to open
a bag and graze later at night than it is to cook
up some healthy vegetables.

The point is, we inherit a lot of bad habits
from our parents… such as portion size,
cooking with grease/lard/butter, and being
told to finish your entire plate.

Breaking free from parental bad habits can
cause estranged strife in any family.

When I used to go to a bodybuilding gym
there was teasing I'd overhear about lifting
light weights. I always wanted to tell them, *"I
train for tone, endurance and balance… not*

*for mass*." In other words, their goals were not my goals. Don't confuse the two.

It's not about strength; it's about control.

So get your head in the game.

It's not about them.
It's about you.

Yet it pays to remember that spot reductions don't work. Either you lose weight over ALL areas of your body... or you don't. That's where toning is better than being able to lift super-heavy weights. For me, my goal is keeping my metabolism high... not low. That's how overall weight-loss goals get achieved. Remember, you're trying to create an overall healthy lifestyle which incorporates greater degrees of exercise each day.

I've seen morbidly obese people who would hit the health club and lift ten times the weight I would, but they'd do it for ten seconds and take a three minute break in between sets. Meanwhile, I'd lift small weights for three minutes and only take ten second breaks. Whose metabolism do you think was higher in that scenario?

## *Chapter Six*

## *Outdoor Chores*

*"Not enough people weed their garden."*
That's a saying I coined in 1997.

Pruning… enables vertical growth over horizontal expansion.  Like manicured shrubs, do you prune your diet so that your bodily goals arrive?

When the weather is nice, weeding, mowing, sweeping, shoveling, planting… all consume calories.  When the weather is bad, shoveling snow is a great workout.

Seeing the results of your outdoor chores exercises more places than your body.

That metaphor visually applies to how you groom your physique.

Change is a choice.  If you change your routine, are you doing the same amount of work?  That's something to consider.  I once complimented one man for using a new piece of cardio equipment because he would just walk on the treadmill for hours each day.  The problem is, when he did that, he ceased working the same amount and gained weight. So perhaps my compliment in his desire to change things up actually hurt the amount of work he did daily.  In other words, walk the walk in order to talk the talk.

Yet when summertime rolls around, I find it hard to exercise inside a gym.  I'd rather be outside... walking, weeding, pruning, raking, and even taking my dumbbells outside to work out in the sunshine.  The vitamin D does do a body good.  When the sunshine becomes abundant, the seasonal affective disorder (S.A.D) goes into hibernation.

So add those extra outdoor chores to your workout routine.  They all count.

## *Chapter Seven*

## *First On, Last Off*

Being honored to witness someone else's physical transformation helps inspire us all to take it up a notch and create our own transformations too. That's one of the things I've loved about paying for 3-4 months of gym time in January, then taking the summer months off to use the outdoors as my place of exercise, and then coming back to the gym and seeing the various amounts in progress that the regulars have achieved. It inspires.

Yet the premise of this chapter is a fundamental law of how our bodies shed extra pounds. Where we put weight on first is the last place where it will come off. So again, it's like peeling the layers of an onion. For men, belly fat is the last place where our weight will come off. For women, it tends to be the legs and hips where weight first accumulates. Unfortunately, a lot of infomercials try to take advantage of that. For example, in women, when they lose weight, part of the fat that gets shed is from the breasts... so it's a reality that if you're a bit busty, when you lose weight, you'll lose breast size as well since they are made up of fat. It's similar to when I lose weight, and my baseball caps suddenly don't fit because I've even lost fat from the area of my head.

Interval training, super sets, and pushing past the point of muscle exhaustion are ways that bodybuilders use to shed those toughest pounds that are the last to come off. For example, with super sets, you exercise one body part, like legs, and then immediately start doing upper body exercises, and then come back to your legs again, and then going back to your upper body again… all without any rest in between sets. That creates a sense of muscle exhaustion in your legs while your upper body's muscles are resting, and then exhausting the upper body, and immediately going back to the legs which have been resting while doing the upper body exercises. It creates a very efficient work-out in a short amount of time. That's my priority when I hit the health club – exercise efficiency.

Exercise permutations and variations (shocking the muscles past plateaus) are other ways that bodybuilders use to maximize their workouts. That's because muscle confusion works. It's all about doing variations of exercises so the muscles never know what's coming next. It pushes you in ways your muscles aren't accustomed to doing. It works.

While stepping on the scale often allows you to analyze how much effort it takes to burn off what you eat and the toll midnight snacks can take, the real results of your muscle building can confuse you into believing that you've actually gained fat when really what you've done is create calorie-consuming muscle… because muscle weighs more than fat. This happened to me when I first started getting back into an exercise regimen. I started at 234 pounds with a body-mass-index of 34% fat. Then I went up to 245 pounds and got my body-mass-index (BMI) measured again one year later, and my BMI was 24%. So even though the scale said that I'd gained weight, I'd lost 10% of my body fat while gaining the appropriate amount of muscle that made my pants fit a lot better than before.

That's where I learned about the beer belly blues… where I can't see my own shoes. The moral of the story is that you don't drink your calories. You should eat them instead.

Now here's a Beer Toast I came across during a walk through a mall recently:

*To nights*
*I won't remember*
*With friends*
*I can't forget*

A moment of levity often breaks the monotony of any dull routine.

So here's another: Bumper sticker slogan to inspire: "*I am a leaf on the wind… watch how I soar.*"

Now I'll end this chapter with an example. There's one girl at gym that went from ripped to fat to ripped again for bodybuilding competitions each summer… and then wondered why she didn't take first place. To me, she gained the winter weight on purpose in order to have the raw material to build bigger, more massive muscles. That's how bodybuilders like to put on mass. They have to have the raw material in place… sort of like a sculptor putting more clay on the potter's wheel… so you can mold it into shape. The problem for the competition is that she didn't get ripped enough… due to the winter weight she purposely gained. So her technique was to see-saw as she alternated between training and packing on pounds. The metaphor is like in golf: *"Drive for show; putt for dough."* Drive for show equates with being able to build massive muscles. Putt for dough implies the fact that chiseled abs sell when it comes to competitions. Also though, I suppose all the excruciating work she put in to train for competitions needed its time of rest afterwards. After all, it's the silences that help make the music flow, right?

## *Chapter Eight*

## *1-Minute Workout*

The new 7-minute workout fad – key:
intensity. Yet the trainer who created it
mentioned how 7 minutes really isn't enough.
Really, he said, you need three 7-minute
sessions. The same is true with doing 60 1-
minute workouts. The key is to just do them.

So tell yourself that you're just gonna
exercise for a minute. And then try to do
those one-minute sessions spaced all
throughout the day. You'd be amazed what
getting in the exercise groove does. It
perpetuates more. The hard part is often just
starting.

Often, it's the endorphins that keep exercise
fun… instead of feeling like you're
trudging… or slogging through the mud.

It creates something *"achievable"* everyday
for everyone. It starts a daily structure of
stealing moments to stretch, strengthen, and
live stronger. It fuels the little train that could
– telling yourself: *"C'mon, you can do it!"* It
provides a new lease on life. Keep in mind
that full range of motion is important… as is
velocity of exercise for power.

"*Commit to get fit*" – commit to 1 minute of exercise every hour you're awake and see how you feel. It creates an "*inch-pebbles vs. mile-stones*" philosophy to your life. You see, one manager once told a group of us engineers that if you think of completing many small tasks as achieving "*inch-pebbles*," you can eventually arrive at your desired "*mile-stones*" much easier. In other words, achieving small tasks towards an overall bigger task provides a greater degree of consistent momentum that gets the job done. Remember that muscle burns fat... so the moral is that it's better to be sore than soaked.

Light, cheap weights do the trick if you use them enough. And that's the whole point of my one-minute workouts that you fit into your routine all throughout the day.

For example, yoga, stretching, and flexibility increase blood flow via all those stretches. My former boss achieved great waistline reduction results this way so he provides the proof in the pudding that stretching alone does work. He just does in a lot, and it has increased his mindfulness towards exercise. He lost 30-40 pounds this way.

The thing to keep in mind is that bad form robs you for maximizing the time and effort you put in... range of motion is crucial, and it is often the biggest mistake I see.  As the saying goes, "*Safety is no accident.*"

Now here's another quote from the Powerhouse Gym newsletter I receive that describes interval training cardio.  It's great food for thought.

*"Basically, you are alternating periods of very high and low intensity. For example, if you are running a track you may sprint for 30 seconds followed by doing a walk for 90 seconds. You repeat this 6-8 times. This takes you way out of your comfort zone and makes your body have to recover afterwards. Recovery takes extra energy.*

*So, mix it up! Keep your cardio fun! Mix some interval training, some speed cardio, and strength training. This is one of the best combinations for weight loss. And a lot less monotonous than day after day on the treadmill. When exercise is NOT boring, you're more likely to keep up with it!"*

## *Chapter Nine*

## *No Sweat Exercises*

Medical studies show that there is a sitting-obesity connection… too much sitting is dangerous to your waistline. This is one reason many offices have stand-up desks now… simply because standing promotes a healthier boost to your metabolism.

So find an excuse to do a lap around the inner-rings of your corporate corridors.

Increase your walking by investing in *"Pedometer Awareness"* where it's reported that our bodies are most efficient with the walking of the 10,000 steps we need each day. You might be surprised when you have a pedometer… which counts each and every step you make… how much walking it really does take to reach 10,000 steps. Yet this is where fitting in sixty one-minute-workouts to each day does add up to healthier totals.

For example, don't underestimate the importance of multi-tasking at work… while you're waiting for a computer to boot, do some stretches to get the blood flowing. If you're waiting at the copy machine, consider doing some toe-raises for your calves and balance.

The whole principle of cubicle cardio is to avoid getting sweaty in situations where it's frowned upon (for example, I got fired from a gym & exercise equipment retail store for using their exercise equipment when no customers were around). So if you still want to maintain your workout, boost your metabolism, and increase blood flows… then you have to do it a bit on the down-low. It's kind of like being an undercover exerciser. That's because the corporate culture often frowns upon anything that isn't work-related. Yet that shouldn't stop you from walking the stairs instead of taking the elevator. That shouldn't stop you from stretching a bit or taking a lap around the cave of cubicles.

Sometimes it's about stealin' moments to stretch and strengthen – by being conscious of minor workout habits – such as the catcher's squat, Kegels, isometrics and crunches, ballet dips for inner thighs, straight-leg toe-touches (limber hamstrings), calf stretches while climbing stairs, and walking on your toes (to work on balance).

When I've fit these kinds of minor fitness techniques to my overall day, I became surprised coming home from work, relaxing, and realizing how truly sore some of my muscles were due to my workplace workout routine in the nooks and crannies of the day.

Another thing to keep in mind is that speed matters when it comes to fast-twitch muscle growth... which tends to atrophy with age... but also is a more efficient use of your exercise time. From physics, power equals mass times acceleration so the speed at which you do these cubicle cardio routines does matter, but it gives you greater bang for the buck with the fast-twitch-muscle fat-burning speed workout techniques. In other words, the speedier you do the exercises, the more efficient your benefits.

Another thing is that there are pedestrian benefits to walking and taking the time to stop and smell the roses. That's because the proper pace of thinking for the human mind is 2 MPH (miles per hour) – where walking is the correct pace of thinking. It entices flow.

Then there's the destination-driven exercise – which is exercise serves a purpose – a goal to reach and arrive... instead of just walking the endless treadmill to nowhere.

Think about any scene in any movie... its purpose is some sort of transformation.

So park far away in good weather (save money on parking for pricy events)... exception: parking in a bad neighborhood. This is a case where parking nearby with security matters. One time, when I went to a Chicago Blackhawks hockey game, my friend parked on the street instead of parking in the stadium's pay-to-park lot. When we came out from the game, we discovered our rear window had been smashed, the trunk's lock was jimmied, and all of our bags were forever stolen. So sometimes, you want to be aware of your surroundings when deciding where to park for extra exercise.

The main goal is to focus on what you can still do (not on what you can't do) – add one new thing (new muscles improve and your brain gets out of a rut). Another idea is to work out next to someone working out hard with intensity because research shows extra effort is contagious. It's like an exercise osmosis that gets absorbed by just being in the near proximity to someone who is training really hard.

Now here's a lesson that I learned from my dog… it's the importance of getting fresh air (refined air vs. "*pure*" air) – it brings you one step closer to nature – awaken & refresh.

The issue is not upsetting the balance of the other employees being jealous of your stepping out to awaken and refresh (easier in corporate settings) – especially in start-up companies – badges that monitor entry and exit times also may prohibit outdoor walks. The point is not to get sweaty while still increasing your metabolism.

Take advantage of those lulls in the day.
Utilize them to increase your overall health.

Some people always say "*tomorrow*" – no,
<u>today</u> and <u>now</u> are your most important
moments.  As Henry Ford is quoted as saying,
"*You can't build a reputation on what you're
going to do.*"  So as Nike says, "*Just do it.*"
Commit to get fit.  Fit happens.

## *Chapter Ten*

## *Break-Ups, Rejection, and Fitness*

Now here's an article I was asked to write for an exercise blog for a female bodybuilder who models and is a spokeswoman for fitness supplements. Its topic revolved around the break-up of a relationship and how it affects our fitness and training regimen.

*I've been told I play better when I'm angry.*

*Having an axe to grind... to prove someone Wrong...*

*...is often the difference between the Winners and Losers in Life.*

*Coping with rejection... even if we're competing for Mr. or Ms. Olympia... never is Easy.*

*I've been told that you can either be Right... or you can be Happy... not Both. It doesn't go both ways.*

*It's one of those Conservation of Energy things. The product of the Gain and the Bandwidth is always a Constant.*

*The whole point that is the most frustrating is that we can try and train for something... so hard... so long... so gruelingly... only to get rejected... only to Lose... or did We?*

*In all honesty... it may be a Blessing in Disguise.*

*You just don't know it quite Yet.*

*Someday in your future... after you've gained weight, gotten off the workout routine, lost the scholarship you felt was "the Golden Ticket," not gotten selected for "the Team," become complacent, grown lazy... sometimes, those are the Silences that enable your Music to Flow.*

*That's the essence of Oprah's "A-Ha Moments" which she raves about 24-7.*

*It's about - decades from now - you'll receive a Cosmic Wink...*

*...letting you know that God was actually Lookin' Out.*

*You just \*thought\* it was a form of Rejection.*

*Actually, it was a Pull when you were Pushin'.*

*It was a "not now" when you could've sworn it was "ASAP."*

*The whole point to keep in mind is that Life still goes on... even after the Page is Turned.*

*Chapters in our Life come... chapters in our Life go. The Key... is knowing their Arrival and Departure.*

*When it comes to training... it's the Silences that help the music to flow... for our muscles to Grow... Strong.*

*If we didn't put spaces in-between the words we write…*

*…they'dallbecomeabunchofgoobledygookthat'dbe hardtoRead.*

*Thus… to be a Man or Woman of All Seasons… you must know when to Hibernate… and when to Bloom.*

*And Voila… in that transformational Emergence… you realize that the Sky to Fly offers plenty of Room.*

*Rooms to grow… rooms to know.*
*That in you is the seed.*
*Of all you'll really need.*
*To become the person…*
*…you need to Be.*

*May your Life's Emergences be -*
*Transformational - and Real.*

*Brian Shell*

## *Chapter Eleven*

## *Personal Trainers – Kickstart Your Routine*

After years of training on my own, it was interesting to see the results of how a personal training session justified a jumpstart in my training techniques.

When I took those two months off and then resigned a four-month package at my gym, they offered two free personal training sessions. Free is always nice to me.

One of the things I enjoyed most was being pushed into the red... to sweat... profusely.

With a lot of old joint injuries from all the mileage I've put on my body, it's always a concern because I've seen my share of trainers train newbies way, way too hard... which also almost sets them up for failure. They get _so_ sore afterwards. Then they don't want to go back. Yet for a seasoned and salty ol' gym rat, a good kickstart to the ol' ticker may be just what the doctor ordered to take your training to levels beyond the norm.

Training in close proximity with a professional... be careful to chose a trainer who has the sense not to wear too many scents. Too much cologne or perfume is a hindrance, and one of the trainers I've worked out with liked to wear way too much… a headache.

One of the frustrations I've heard echoed from those who do use trainers is that sometimes, they get injuries they don't feel they would have gotten had they not been *"pushed into the red"* by someone who was trying to teach them new training methods. That's one the issues with age… our minds strong… it's our bodies that can be weak. They become brittle with age and atrophy. So when someone has us do something outside our normal training comfort zone, injury often rears its ugly head. Sigh…

Trainers do come in handy though when it comes to someone to be accountable to.

Accountability is often a good motivator to do the work that is exercise.

I even heard of one trainer who has her clients email her each day to tell her what they did today to achieve their fitness goals. Now, that's accountability. Yet it's also coming clean to a person who values your ability to achieve the physical appearance you desire. They cheerlead. They advise. They encourage when you have no one else to encourage you to do the exercise your body needs on a daily basis. Trainers do have value.

Personally, I'm one who has read enough "*Muscle & Fitness*" magazines to know my way around the gym pretty well, but when I've worked out with trainers, I realize that they push me beyond my typical comfort zone of training. That can be a good thing.

## *Chapter Twelve*

## *Final Thoughts about Food and Exercise*

Be conscious about being health conscious

Make it a lifestyle... make it a habit

Life is a marathon, not a sprint. If you like to burn the candle twice as bright, be prepared to conserve your inner reserve later in life so as not to burn out too fast and too soon.

Weights-first/cardio-after is the most efficient philosophy for burning fat. So if you have a short amount of time to exercise, train by lifting weights... even if they're only two or three pound dumbbells that you take a few minutes lifting with all kinds of little exercises as it burns calories long after you're done due to having to rebuild and grow stronger.

Studies have shown that attitude, determination, and intensity do factor into getting better scores on IQ tests too. So remember the slogan: No pain, no gain.

If there's one word I want you to remember from reading this book – *Consistency.*

Consistency translates to *dependability*, and in a long life, that turns into long-term health, strength, and wisdom.  Smart choices are *right* choices.

If you stay consistent over a lifetime, people will trust you.

Don't buy your body, earn it.  So grow your reputation by being accountable... not only to yourself... but to the others who surround you.  Endurance is one of the side-benefits.

Ask yourself, what's more inherently satisfying?  A fortune that falls into your lap or one you take the time to earn?  Think about it... if you won the lottery for millions of dollars, would it mean as much as if you earned through hard work and dedicated passion from following a dream?

So supplement your daily workout with inch-pebbles of exercise, and then you can meet your overall body-image mile-stones.

The fact is... once you gain momentum... you know you're gettin' there.  You <u>do</u> eventually arrive at your body's appearance destination.  So know what you want to achieve because if you don't know your destination, how will you ever know when you reach it?  Give yourself daily goals you <u>can</u> accomplish.

You <u>can</u> change... learn the habit of exercising often.

Do a little… a lot of times a day.

You can do it.

Get out of your comfort zone… try new things.  Add new routines to your day.

Focus on mindful actions… not mindless patterns.

Recently I passed by a church sign echoing the sentiments of today's hectic society: "*If it feels like life's spinning, don't worry, you're just on God's potter's wheel.*"

Whatever happens, don't give up.  Deferred joys purchased through sacrifice are often the sweetest.  Remember to try to find your cure rather than using a band-aid as cover.

Hard work is just that: hard work.  But the inner smile of earned rewards?  Priceless.

## eBooks by the Author:
## Brian Shell
PassionHeroDotCom

Detour
Gratitude Miles
All Men Are Dogs
Making a Masterpiece
A Prodigal Son Returns
Single Mom Soul – Spring
Single Mom Soul – Summer
Single Mom Soul – Autumn
Single Mom Soul – Winter
The Chip
Oprah and I
Mind Games
Here & There
Facebook Diaries
Dessert First Diet
Start My Heart Art
American Romance
Love Poems from the Heart
Texas Hold'em Tournament Tactics
Shastras – Received Wisdom about Right
Conduct
Pre-Celebrity Jesus – The Man Before the
Messiah
A Juxtaposition of Idiosyncrasies
Up from the Snakepit
Teenage Jesus
Distortions